Health Benefits of Coconut Oil

By Muhamad Usman

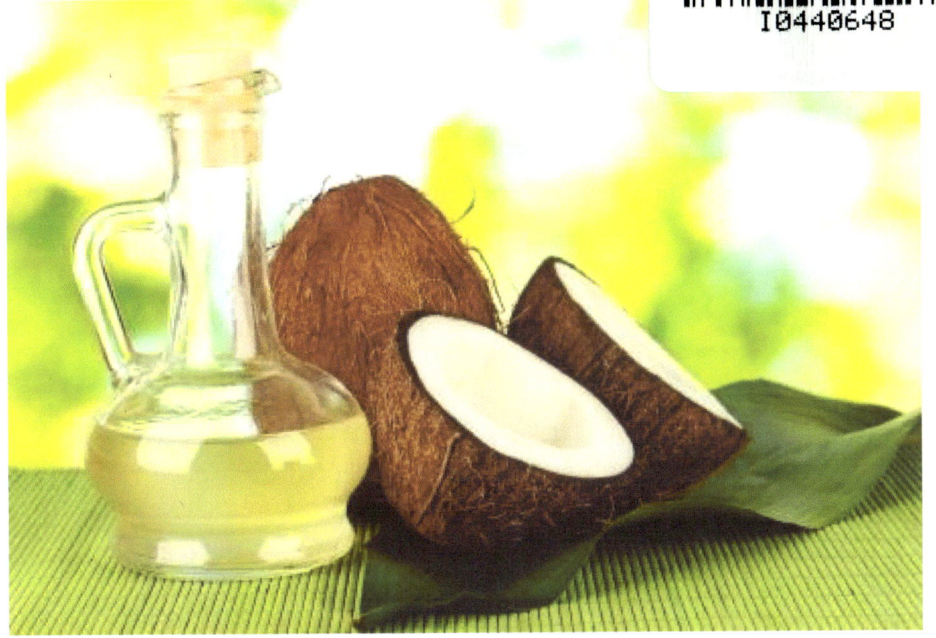

Health Learning Series

Mendon Cottage Books

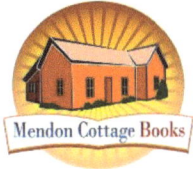

JD-Biz Publishing

Disclaimer

The information is this book is provided for informational purposes only. It is not intended to be used and medical advice or a substitute for proper medical treatment by a qualified health care provider. The information is believed to be accurate as presented based on research by the author.

The contents have not been evaluated by the U.S. Food and Drug Administration or any other Government or Health Organization and the contents in this book are not to be used to treat cure or prevent disease or mental illness.

The author or publisher is not responsible for the use or safety of any diet, procedure or treatment mentioned in this book. The author or publisher is not responsible for errors or omissions that may exist.

Warning

The Book is for informational purposes only and before taking on any diet, treatment or medical procedure it is recommended to consult with your primary care provider.

Our books are available at

1. Amazon.com
2. Barnes and Noble
3. Itunes
4. Kobo
5. Smashwords
6. Google Play Books

Table of Contents

Preface

There are dozens of cooking oils used around the world but few can match the health benefits of coconut oil.

For a long time, coconut oil has been wrongly advertised as an unhealthy food product because of its high unsaturated fat content in order to promote other cooking oils such as canola. The common complaints against coconut oil were elevated cholesterol levels, risk of heart and brain disorders, etc.

Today, research has revealed that coconut oil, although comprising of 90% saturated fats, is quite safe for consumption and contrary to what was advertised, has dozens of health benefits of its own. From being a natural cooking oil that is delicious and having a high smoke point, to a healer of several serious diseases and preventer of a similar number, coconut oil is indeed a blessing of nature that has been misrepresented for a long time.

This book aims to educate the reader on the health benefits of coconut oil and enable them to take full advantage of this healthy commodity in their lives so that they can reap all the health benefits of the oil and avoid any side effects that it may cause.

Getting Started

Chapter # 1: Intro

Before going into the health benefits of coconut oil, this book will provide a short introduction to those who are unfamiliar with it.

Coconut oil is primarily recognized as an edible vegetable oil just like canola, olive or corn oil. Extracted from the meat / kernel of full grown coconuts collected from the coconut palm that botanists call *Cocos nucifera.* It is largely made of fat: comprising of ninety percent saturated, six percent unsaturated and three percent polyunsaturated fat. This extremely high fat content has been used to over advertise it as an unhealthy food product in the past few decades but the truth is far from it.

Unlike other fatty food products containing large quantities of saturated / unsaturated fats, coconut oil's main constituents are medium chain fatty acids or MCFAs. The saturated fat portion of the oil makes it stable to thermal decomposition and allows it to be stored for a long number of time.

Apart from being a healthy and tasty cooking oil, coconut oil has become famous of its ability to heal various conditions, fight inflammation and boost metabolism by the action of its MCFAs. It has transformed from a sidelined cooking oil to the wonder of the dietary world because of recent research which has revealed its ability to perform miracles such as weight loss, reduces hair loss, fight eczema and enhance physical performance of the person who consumes it in a balanced manner.

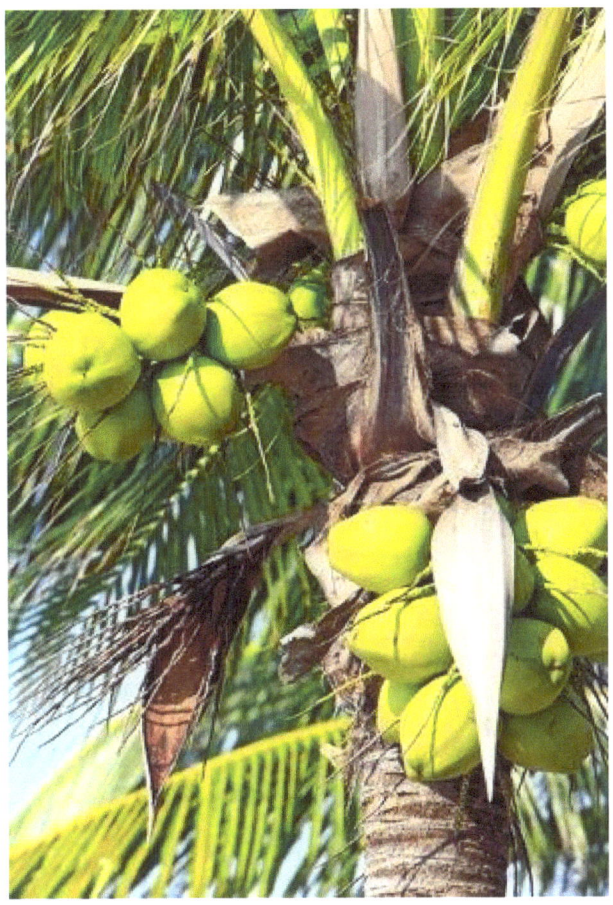

Chapter # 2: Methods of production

There are many ways by which coconut oil can be obtained from the coconut kernel. The primary division is between the 'dry' and 'wet' processes used for the extraction of the oil.

Dry process:

In dry processing, the meat of the coconut has to be removed from its shell and dried under a heat source such as fire, the sun or a kiln. The end product of this drying procedure is 'copra' or dried coconut.

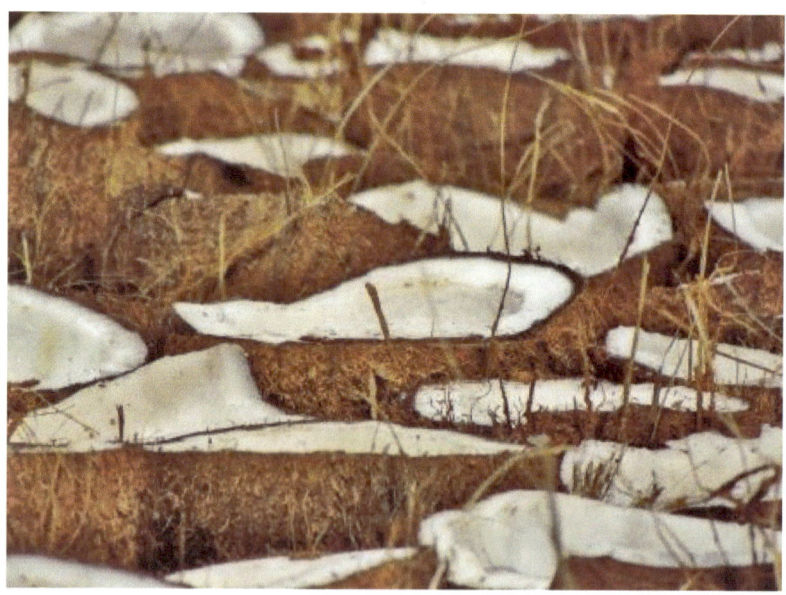

This 'copra' is combined with solvents which yields coconut oil along with a mash rich in both protein and fiber. However, the mash's quality makes it unfit for human consumption so it is fed to cattle such as cows and buffalo. The protein mixed with the mash cannot be separated and so has to go with it as cattle feed. Also, a percentage of the oil present in the copra is lost during extraction.

Wet process:

The wet process is another technique for the extraction of coconut oil and uses raw coconut instead of dried copra. The protein content of the coconut is used to emulsify the oil and water. The main issue is the extraction of the oil from the emulsion that has been created. In the past, boiling for a long period of time used to be the preferred method for separating the oil from the emulsion but this caused discoloration of the oil and was uneconomical. Today, centrifuges combined with techniques such as exposure to thermal extremes, acids, enzymes, electrolysis, salt, shockwaves etc. are used. In spite of the fact that technology has progressed a lot since the early days of wet process extraction, it still has a yield lower than the dry process and is quite costly because of the equipment and energy required to make it work.

The oil making process can be enhanced by using properly harvested coconuts that have matured well. Coconut oil is dissolved in hexane to boost the oil yield by up to ten percent compared to simple extraction by expellers and rotary mills. Afterwards, it is refined to eliminate specific fatty acids that may shorten its shelf life. Shelf life is boosted by additional techniques such as choosing copra with a low moisture content, regulating the amount of moisture in the oil too, and also by adding citric acid / salt to oil that has been heated to around one-forty Celsius degrees.

Virgin coconut oil is a special kind of coconut oil that is made from raw coconut meat, milk or deposit.

RBD:

'Refined, bleached, and deodorized' oil is made from dried copra that is put in a hydraulic press combined with extra heat. Practically all the oil present in the copra is extracted by this technique.

However, the crude coconut oil that has just been extracted cannot be consumed as it is unrefined and may contain contamination. Further heat and filtration is done to make it fit for human consumption.

High quality coconut oil may also be extracted by the action of enzymes. RBD oil has a complete lack of coconut flavor or scent and is used for cooking, processing food, cosmetics, industry and in medicine.

Hydrogenation:

RBD oil may processed additionally to create hydrogenated coconut oil that has a higher melting point. Coconut oils that have not been hydrogenated sometimes tend to melt esp. in warmer locales. Hydrogenation allows coconut oil products to remain solid in warmer climates.

Fractionation:

Fractionation allows specific MCFAs to be extracted from the whole of the coconut oil so they can be utilized for special purposes. For instance, Lauric acid is an especially useful fatty acid present in the oil that has a lot of value in industry and medicine.

Chapter # 3: Types of coconut oil

The main distinction between coconut oils is made on the basis of whether they are refined or not.

Refined coconut oil is made from copra. The main product that falls under this category is coconut oil that has been manufactured under the RBD process detailed above. The RBD process makes the oil extracted from copra fit for human consumption by removing any impurities present in it.

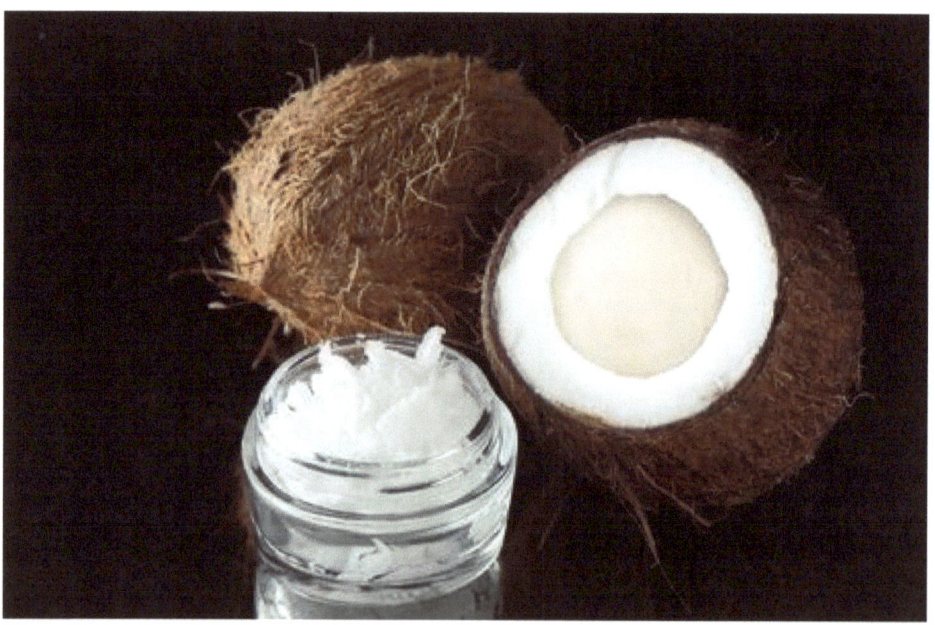

Refined coconut oil, as previously mentioned, is tasteless and odorless making it ideal for deep fried foods because of its high smoke point. Its nutritional value is slightly less than that of virgin or unrefined coconut oil.

The majority of coconut oils present in the market are refined but their quality varies a good deal. Try to obtain non-hydrogenated, good quality oil from a reliable vendor. Make sure that it has been refined by natural and non-chemical processes.

The main advantage of refined oil is that it is cheaper and its fat content enables it to be used as a great bath oil / natural body wash / moisturizer.

Unrefined coconut oil is otherwise known as 'virgin' / 'extra-virgin' coconut oil that is obtained by pressurizing raw coconut under a hydraulic press without any chemical interference. Its flavor ranges from mild to intense depending on the amount of heat provided during the extraction process.

Quality unrefined coconut oil will have a light coconut taste and aroma. The difference between virgin and extra virgin varieties is more of a marketing ploy and both varieties are superior to refined coconut oil.

Chapter # 4: Why is coconut oil so healthy?

Coconut oil owes much of its potency as a healthy food product because of lauric acid, a fatty acid present in coconut oil that has astonishing health boosting attributes. Lauric acid is well known for antimicrobial properties that strengthen the human immune system. And since almost half of coconut oil is comprised of this fatty acid, consumption of coconut oil is a healthy practice.

The body converts lauric acid in to a compound called monolaurin which enables coconut oil to treat conditions such as candida, measles and hepatitis C. Interestingly, another source of this compound is mother's milk which is another clear indication of just how healthy coconut oil is.

The reason why coconut oil is not harmful like other fatty foods is because its composition consists primarily of medium chain fatty acids that are relatively small in length and can be broken down and absorbed by the human digestive and transformed into energy. This is pretty much what happens with glucose minus the sudden increase in insulin levels. Other fatty foods usually comprise of long chain fatty acids or triglycerides that the body finds hard to digest which is why they get stored as fat and what follows is weight gain and a plethora of unhealthy effects.

The MCFAs present in the coconut oil improve our metabolism and encourage the body to utilize stored fat as energy which causes weight loss, lowered risk of type 2 diabetes, boost in energy, quickened healing and also leads to a fortified immune system.

The moisture content of coconut oil makes it great of the skin and helps repair skin tissue.

Chapter # 5: Buying and storing coconut oil

There are dozens upon dozens of brands that sell coconut oil – they're prices vary depending on the coconuts used for extracting the oil, the method of extraction, the packaging quality and the brand. The most expensive brand may not be the best since a lot depends on personal taste and preference but price often indicates production value and top notch ingredients. The best way to decide upon the coconut oil to use at home is to try out a few brands and choose among them based on their taste, effect on health etc.

Some things to keep an eye on when choosing brands include:

Color: Try to purchase coconut oil that is white when solid and transparent when molten. Discoloration indicates a degree of contamination in the production process.

Taste and scent: If you're purchasing virgin coconut oil then it should have a reasonably light coconut taste and aroma – say no to virgin oil that has a roasted or smoked flavor since it has probably been heated excessively and may not retain as many nutrients. If you are purchasing refined coconut oil, you should go for a product that has no taste and no color.

Price: Try buying coconut oil wholesale to save on cash since retail stores often sell coconut oil at high cost which may not get you the best value for money. You needn't worry about the oil going rancid since it can last for at least a year before showing signs of age. Trying out a few different brands initially will help you find the right one.

You can store coconut oil without refrigeration by keeping it away from sunlight – this way, it will last for up to 24 months. Coconut oil usually stays liquid at room temperature and turns into coconut butter when the temperature starts to go down. However, a small amount of heat is enough to change it back into a liquid.

Chapter # 6: Using coconut oil

There are great many ways in which coconut oil can be used at home. It can be used in cooking fried foods, for the nourishment of one's skin, for treating common conditions such as flu and cold or as a disinfectant and healing agent for bruises and cuts.

The recommended dosage of coconut oil for an average adult person is between three and four tablespoons per day. Children require a lower amount and as do those who are new to saturated fats. For instance, if you're switching over from a low fat diet to a high fat one, you should gradually increase your intake of coconut oil to get your body used to the fatty content, otherwise you might experience diarrhea when you start out.

Here are some general tips on how to use coconut oil in your daily life:

As food:

Because of its thermal stability, coconut oil is great for deep frying food in it and garnishing roasts and sauces. Asian cooking in particular benefits greatly from its taste that compliments the overall dish.

It is usually solid at room temperature which makes it a good replacement for butter and margarine in making spreads, baked goods and sweet dishes. A one to one ratio should be used when making the substitution. Examples of dishes that can be made in this way include grain free granola, chocolate truffles, fried meatballs and mayonnaise.

You can also add one or two tablespoons of coconut oil to enhance the flavor of drinks such as shakes, juices and tea. You can even eat frozen coconut oil with a spoon – it tastes more like white chocolate than an oil!

Coconut oil mixed with cacao and honey makes for a great power boosting good that can be eaten before exercise.

For skin- and hair-care:

Coconut oil is an excellent face and body moisturizer that many women use to get rid of stretch marks.

It can also be utilized as a bath oil – four or five tablespoons in a hot tub are all that's required for soft, moist skin after a bath!

Coconut oil can be used to make natural soap, deodorant etc. Massage your scalp with it a couple of hours before taking a shower for healthy, glowing, fizz free hair.

Coconut oil can also be used to treat sunburn and even protect the skin from the sun since it contains SPF4.

It also serves as a natural antibacterial skin rub so you can use it as an aftershave too!

By mixing it with some sugar / salt, you can get a natural exfoliator to get rid of dead skin on your feet.

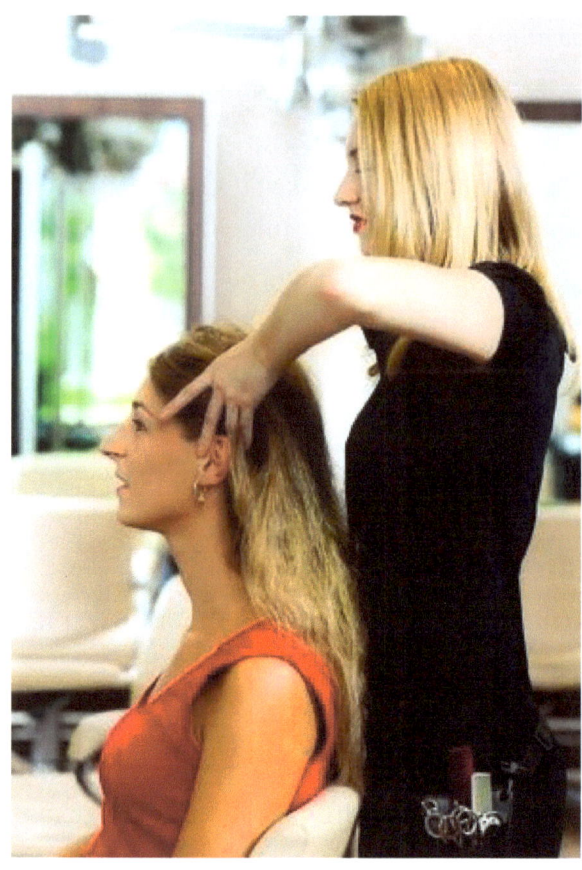

Aside from these uses, it can be used as an anti-lice treatment, healing agent, vapor rub, anti-yeast treatment etc.

With so many uses and so many ways to make coconut oil a part of your life, there is no way to justify not using this healthy food at home. All you need to do is follow the tips and instructions present in this section of the book and you will soon find yourself reaping the many benefits of coconut oil. You needn't worry about its disadvantages so long as you consume it in moderation, according to your diet plan and requirements. Besides, much of the dirt thrown at it has been disproven by research.

Benefits of coconut oil to the brain

Chapter # 7: Protects against neurodegenerative conditions

The human brain requires a continuous source of energy to make it function correctly. As soon as this energy stream gets interrupted, neurons in the brain start to die out. The immediate effects of this condition are headaches, exhaustion and brain fog. But in the long run, a lack of energy supply to the brain leads to permanent degeneration of the human brain.

Recent research has indicated towards coconut oils ability to provide brain with a clean fuel source that takes care of all short term and long term effects of energy deprivation on the brain.

The culprit behind the onset of several neurodegenerative disorders is the insulin resistance that occurs in neurons in the central portion of the brain. Insulin is required to provide glucose in the cells – and glucose is the source of energy for these cells. In short – the brain has become diabetic – it is unable to obtain glucose for energy causing the cells to die from a lack of proper nutrition.

Since the brain cannot take in the sugar that body is sending its way, the blood sugar levels in the brain become elevated – these heightened levels of sugar are toxic for the brain's neurons since it leads to increased oxidative stress and neuron damage. This toxic blood sugar level coupled with the lack of nutrients for the brain cells causes something of a death storm in the brain.

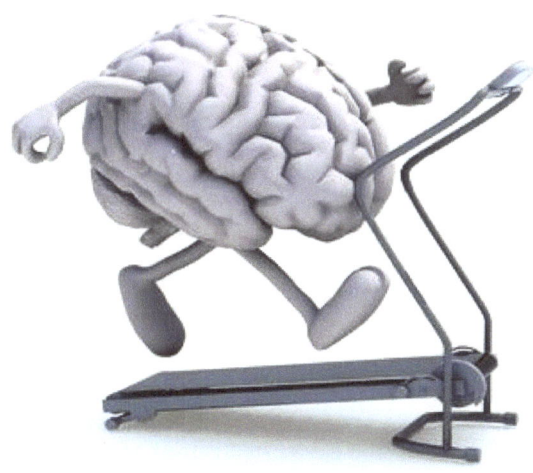

Coconut oil is one of nature's best sources of medium chain triglycerides that are essential for proper brain health. These triglycerides are not dealt with in the same way as long chain triglycerides which are digested by the body after being exposed to bile salts produced by the gallbladder.

MCTs go to the liver without any bile breakdown and get converted into ketones that are injected straight into the bloodstream and sent to the brain to be used as an energy source that is both stable and does not carry the same risks as elevated blood sugar levels. Ketones are, in essence, the food source of choice for those effected with neurological disorders such as Alzheimer's, ALS, Parkinson's, Multiple Sclerosis etc.

Dr. Mary Newport has shown that ketones can aid the newborn's brain in recovering from brain death caused by oxygen deprivation. Research conducted on dogs has shown that dogs that consumed MCTs in their diet had better age related memory performance because the MCTs aided in the release of omega 3 fatty acids that are required to form memory centers in the brain.

Such solid research is indicative of the fact that those who want to prevent themselves from becoming mentally disabled in their later years should consume coconut oil on a daily basis so that their brain stays in mint condition even as they grow old. Those who already suffer from diabetes or some neurological condition should in take more coconut oil than the average recommended amount of three to four tablespoons daily. This will provide them with a clean energy source without increasing the sugar content in their bloodstream.

Benefits of coconut oil to the body

Chapter # 8: Fights heart disease

Coconut oil has been identified as a potent new weapon in the fight against heart disease. This is quite surprising since coconut oil was previously advertised as a promoter of heart disease. As it turns out, consuming liberal quantities of coconut oil can actually bring down the risk of a heart attack!

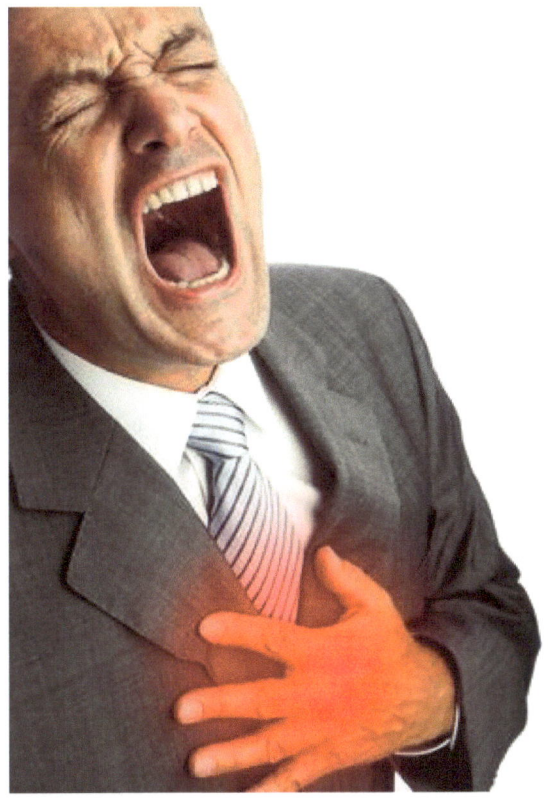

The MCFAs present in coconut oil are responsible for bringing down the risk of heart attack even though they were slandered as saturated fats in the previous years. As it turns out, MCFAs are completely different in the way they are handled by our digestive system compared to long chain fatty acids which are harmful for the body.

The main argument against coconut oil had been that it increases the cholesterol level of the blood. The truth is that it does raise the cholesterol level but this raise is in HDL cholesterol which is actually good for the overall cholesterol profile. This good cholesterol protects against heart disease. The total blood cholesterol is the collective HDL and LDL (bad cholesterol) levels combined and does not prove to be a good indicator of heart disease. The correct chance of heart disease can be obtained by the ratio between LDL and HDL and since coconut oil improves the HDL levels, the ratio declines and as does the risk of heart attack.

Many well reputed studies have illustrated the fact those people who consume coconut oil as a part of their natural diet have a very low occurrence of heart attacks and related conditions.

Even in the '70s and '80s when the campaign against coconut oil was at its peak, its consumption was seen to be related with many signs indicating a healthy heart such as better cholesterol readings, reduced body fat, decreased mortality rate, lowered blood clotting tendency, lessened number of uncontrolled free radicals present in the cell, better antioxidant quantity in the cells and reduced occurrence of heart attacks. This clearly establishes that coconut oil is good for the heart or at the very least, contrary to what was propagated in the media, it is neutral. But this wasn't all the research found. A new property of coconut oil was discovered that made it a promising candidate for a strong weapon against heart conditions.

Heart disease occurs due to the hardening of the arteries which occurs in the form of plaque on their lining. It is thought to be caused by injury that occurs to the lining of the arteries which may be caused by toxic compounds, bacteria, viruses or free radicals. These agents cause irritate and inflame the artery lining causing the development of scar tissue on it. Whenever platelets encounter an injury in the artery, they tend to clot and bond to the damaged area which ultimately results in an intricate mixture of scar tissue, calcium, cholesterol, triglycerides and platelets that is what is otherwise called plaque of the arteries. If plaque starts to develop in the coronary artery that supplies the heart with bloods, it leads to coronary heart disease.

Atherosclerosis or hardening of the arteries has been found to be linked with low level infections particularly bacterial and viral infections. This is the reason why so many people who are apparently fit suffer from heart attacks all of a sudden. Although there are other causes of heart disease, this is a significant contributor. There are numerous cases which point in favor of this discovery including cases where patients suffering from chlamydia, herpes or CMV has elevated chances of heart attack. Chlamydia in particular has been found to particularly good at instigating heart conditions. These microbes stay in the body indefinitely and may damage the artery lining based on how poor the person's immune system is at handling them.

Heart disease may be treated with antibiotics according to the studies above, however these can only deal with bacteria. The good news is that an MCFA present in coconut oil will kill all malign microbes that may lead to heart disease. MCFAs are well known and potent germ killers that will help you take care of infection and also the resultant heart risk it poses.

Another strong indication towards the heart beneficent effects of coconut oil is the fact that countries such as Sri Lanka and regions of India, where coconut oil used to be an integral part of cooking, had very few reports of heart disease but when coconut oil was made notorious to promote other cooking oils in these areas, the number of heart attacks increased.

Today, researchers are once again returning back to the opinion that coconut oil is indeed good for heart health contrary to what was advertised for years because findings indicate that heart attack figures have actually risen since the introduction of other types of cooking oil.

Chapter # 9: Cures candida

Coconut oil has proven to be very effective against candida. It alleviates the painful symptoms of the disease quite effectively. With its ability to prevent loss of moisture, it is very good at preventing the cracking or peeling of skin that is a distinguishing symptom of candida. An important quality of coconut oil is that it cures candida in a gradual manner which allows the body to adjust to the withdrawal symptoms that manifest themselves as candida is being rooted out of the body. The best way to take advantage of coconut oil's candida fighting powers is to start with a moderate dose and increase gradually.

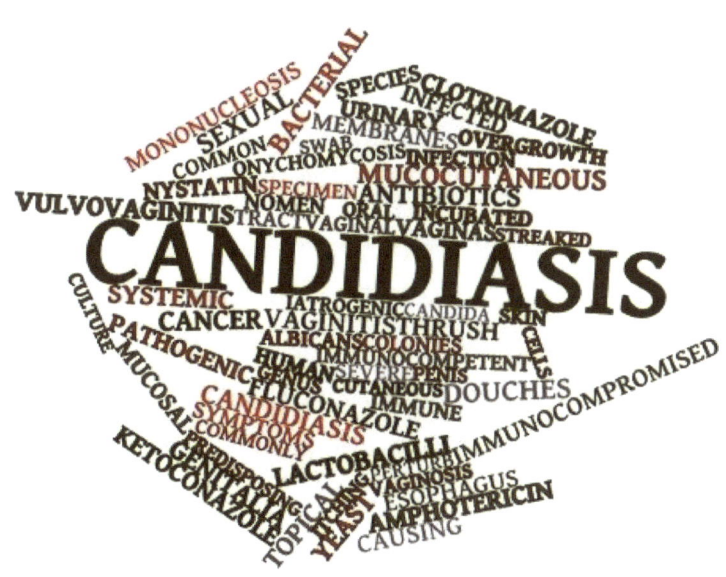

Candida is an extremely troublesome condition that occurs due to the uncontrolled formation of yeast in the stomach. The yeast is known as Candida Albicans. Although this yeast is present in a small quantity in nearly everyone's gut, it doesn't cause anything bad because its growth is contained by the good bacteria in the stomach. If the good bacteria in the stomach get killed off due to some malignant microbes or excessive use of antibiotics then the yeast starts to grow out of proportion leading to the onset of Candida. Furthermore, using laxatives, taking in harmful chemicals, or washing the stomach with lots of medication can lead to the abnormal growth of the yeast leading to Candida.

The symptoms of candida range from infection of the privates, bladder and urinary tract, gut, nose, throat and ear; parched, patched, itchy and peeling skin; internal and external inflammation; upset digestive and excretory systems and unhealthy nails and hair. In Europe and America, where Candida is more common, a large portion of foods involve some yeast culture or fermentation process for their production. These cultures aid the growth of Candida Albicans in the gut.

There are several fatty acids present in coconut oil that negate the effects of these habits and thus prevent the onset of Candida.

For instance, capric acid is an MCFA found in coconut oil that has the ability to fight all sorts of infections including but not limited to fungus. In fact, it is the very same molecule that is present in breast milk so that babies receive protection from infections. Once inside the body, it interacts with enzymes produced by other bacteria to transform itself into a potent infection killer i.e. monocaprin. Controlled use of coconut oil by candida patients has shown the capric acid to be very good at taking care of the yeast.

Aside from capric acid, coconut oil also contains lauric acid, myristic acid, caproic acid and caprylic acid, all of which boast infection killing attributes that help in dealing with candida.

Chapter # 10: Effective against diabetes

Type 2 diabetes:

The general perception about combating type 2 diabetes up until now had been to use prescription drugs but now, researchers and patients alike are cottoning on to the fact that type 2 diabetes can in fact be dealt with through a healthy diet and lifestyle without resorting to medications. Those who were into the alternative health scene knew about this information several years prior to the common public. In fact, there are testimonials as old as over a decade from people who have experienced improvement in their diabetes condition through the use of coconut oil!

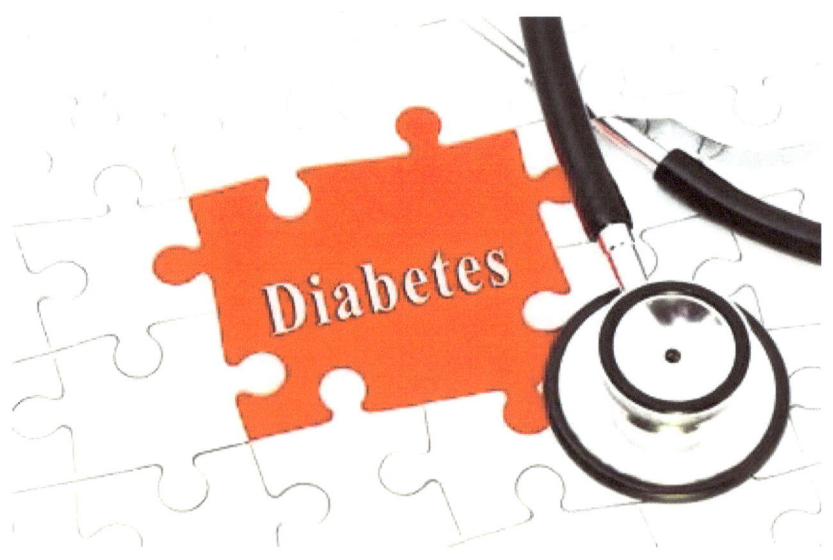

The key to defeating type 2 diabetes through a healthy lifestyle is to limit your intake of refined sugar, carbs and alcohol, and, at the same time, increasing the consumption of good saturated fats and proteins. Most of the people suffering from type 2 diabetes consume foods cooked in oils such as corn and soybean which contain lots of long chain polyunsaturated fats that are quite harmful for someone with diabetes. Replacing these cooking oils with coconut oil that contains healthy saturated fats reduces the hunger pangs that occur frequently otherwise leading to lowered insulin resistance that is the mark of diabetes.

Coconut oil's potential to reduce food cravings is backed by substantial evidence. It promotes thermogenesis and raises the rate of metabolism in the body. Several population studies have been conducted to analyze the effect of coconut oil on human health. For instance, a study conducted in India reached the conclusion that when Indians left their traditional coconut oil and ghee in favor of canola and sunflower oils, their diabetes figures elevated to alarming levels. Similar results were reached in studies that took place in the South Pacific islands.

A study conducted at Australia's Garvan Institute of Medical Research in 2009 showed that a diet containing coconut oil counters the development of 'insulin resistance' in the body. It also prevents fat from getting stored due to the intake of long chain fatty acids. Since insulin resistance and being overweight are serious contributors towards type 2 diabetes, this solidifies the claim that coconut oil is effective against type 2 diabetes.

Chapter # 11: Promotes skin health

Coconut oil has amazing skin enhancing properties too. It has potent moisturizing ability that works with every type of skin including, obviously, dry skin. Mineral oil and coconut oil have a comparable effect on the skin. But since mineral oil can have a negative effect on the skin, coconut oil is the better choice among the two for continuous use as a moisturizer on skin that has a tendency to get dry or flaky.

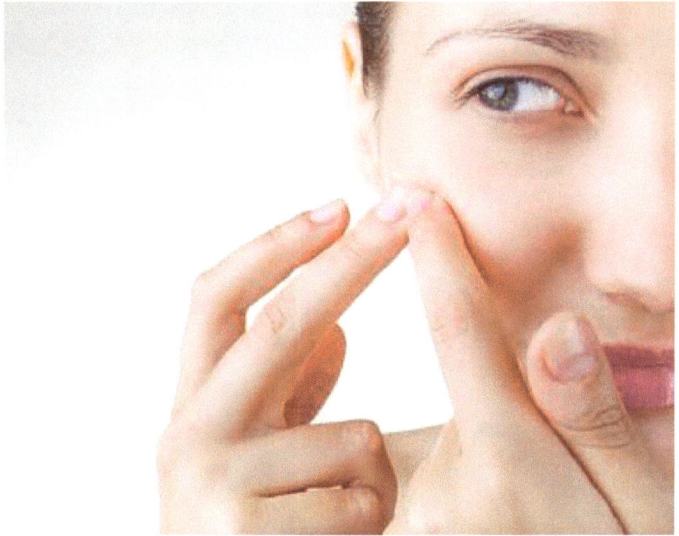

Apart from this, coconut oil has the ability to delay the onset of age effects such as wrinkles and sagging on the skin. Skin conditions such as eczema, psoriasis, dermatitis, etc. are also treatable by coconut oil. These properties of coconut oil to boost skin health are the reason why it is a core ingredient in soaps, creams and lotions. Its antioxidant properties further aid in preventing age effects.

Chapter # 12: Promotes hair health

Coconut oil is on top of the list of natural nutrients for healthy hair. If you want your hair to grow thick and shiny, coconut oil is a must. Unhealthy hair caused by the loss of proteins can be stoppered through the application of coconut oil to the scalp.

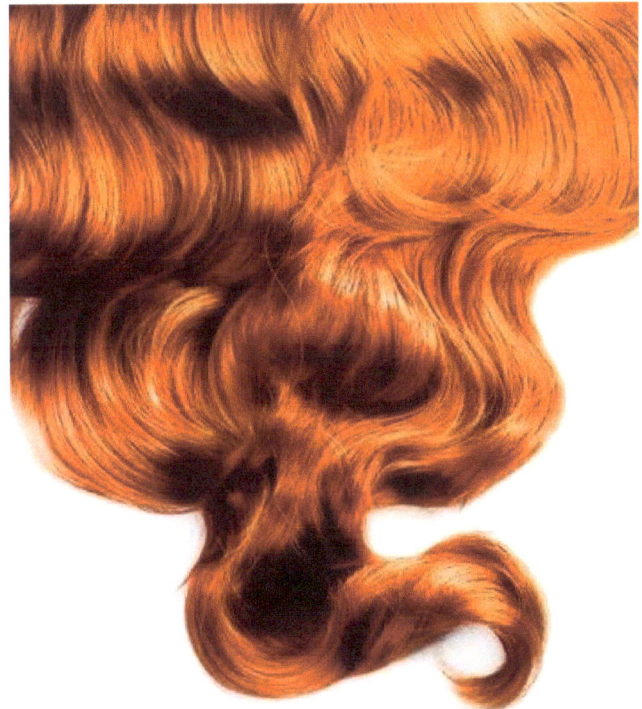

Coconut oil has been used in India for improving hair health since centuries. In fact, it is the habit of many people to massage their scalps with coconut oil after having bathed. It is a great natural hair conditioner and repairs damaged hair by providing the necessary proteins they require. Some studies have shown that hair damage from hygral fatigue can be avoided by applying coconut oil on one's hair.

Coconut oil also takes care of dandruff – even in the most severe cases and even shields from parasites like lice. It is a good idea to use coconut oil regularly to keep your hair in tip top form.

If you need any more convincing, have a look at all the hair care products that boost coconut oil as their major ingredient!

Chapter # 13: Aids digestion

Coconut oil is known to keep the digestive system working in good form when consumed as a cooking oil. It prevents stomach related conditions such as Irritable Bowel Syndrome. It does so because of saturated fats that it contains which are potent germ killers. These saturated fats take care of microbes, bacteria, and fungi etc. that cause stomach disorders. Moreover, coconut oil also aides in the uptake of other nutrients e.g. minerals, vitamins and amino acids.

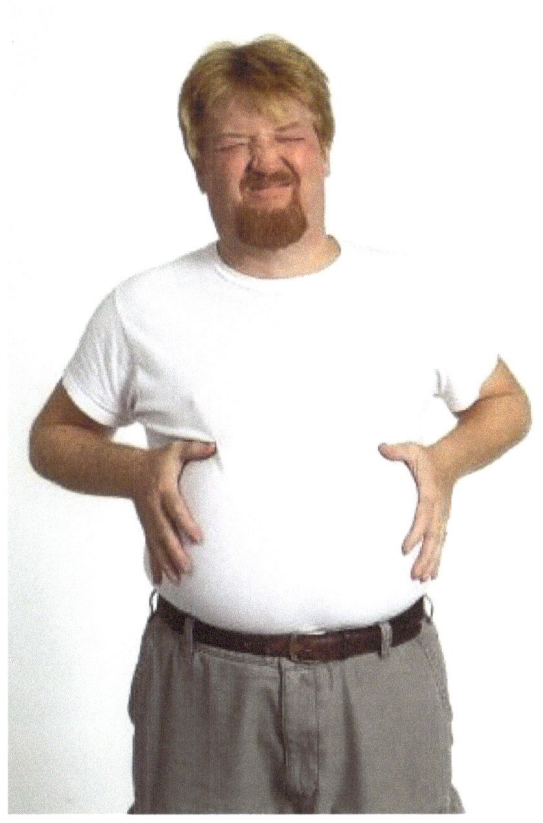

Conclusion

Now that you have come to the end of the book and become awakened to the true nature and potential of coconut oil in terms of its health benefits, you will begin to realize how misguided the mass media can be.

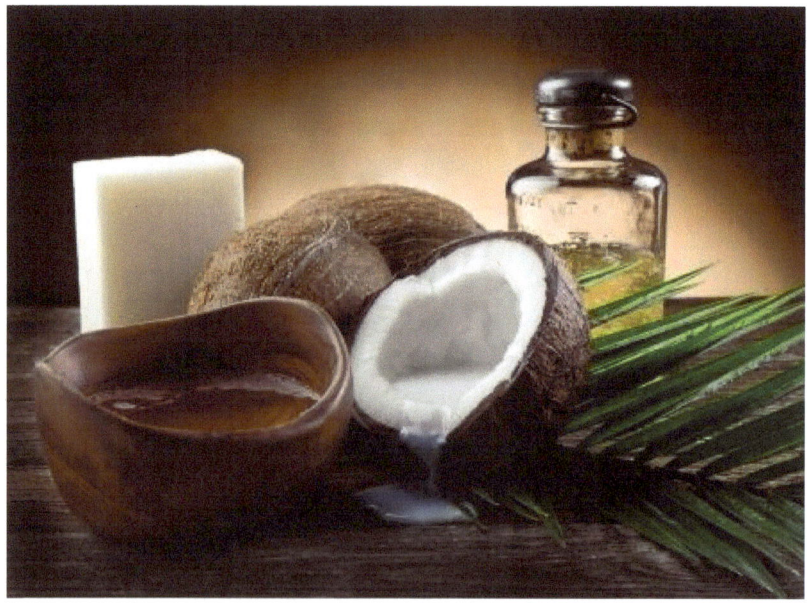

The same media that used to condemn coconut oil and promote other cooking oils today has admitted its mistake and started to promote it as a healthy food item. Its benefits are many and immense and pertain to both the brain and the body and the ease with which it can be incorporated in one's daily life makes it even better.

If you really want to improve your health through healthy living, coconut oil is one of the surest and most profitable first steps you can take.

References

1. http://www.123rf.com/photo_15283076_decanter-with-coconut-oil-and-coconuts-on-green-background.html
2. http://www.123rf.com/photo_8176630_closeup-of-tropical-coconut.html
3. http://www.123rf.com/photo_16296426_opened-cocnut-halves-drying-in-the-sun-before-oil-extraction--central-cocnut-in-focus.html
4. http://www.123rf.com/photo_25785389_natural-coconut-oil-and-coconuts.html
5. http://www.123rf.com/photo_10428056_woman-at-the-hairdresser-getting-a-head-massage-in-the-salon.html
6. http://us.fotolia.com/id/45156048
7. http://us.fotolia.com/id/49672671
8. http://www.123rf.com/photo_16740204_abstract-word-cloud-for-candidiasis-with-related-tags-and-terms.html
9. http://us.fotolia.com/id/39611032
10. http://us.fotolia.com/id/54507728
11. http://www.123rf.com/photo_12632216_red-hair-isolated-on-white.html
12. http://www.123rf.com/photo_3999695_portrait-on-isolated-withe-background-of-a-handsome-expressive-senior.html
13. http://www.123rf.com/photo_9555905_natural-coconut-walnut-oil.html

Author Bio

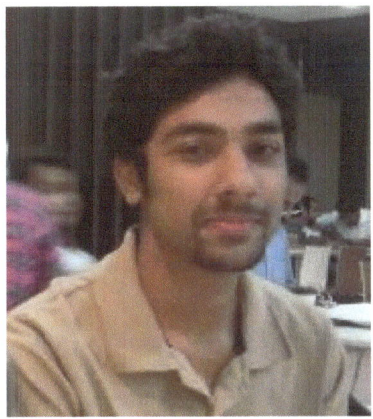

Muhammad Usman is a distinguished medical graduate of Allama iqbal medical college (AIMC). He is a professional writer who has been in the field for more than 4 years. During this time he has produced 10,000+ articles, blogs and eBooks on various niches related to diseases, health, fitness, nutrition and well being. He is a regular contributor to several journals related to medicine and surgery. He is the editor of several journals and newspapers.

Check out some of the other JD-Biz Publishing books

Gardening Series on Amazon

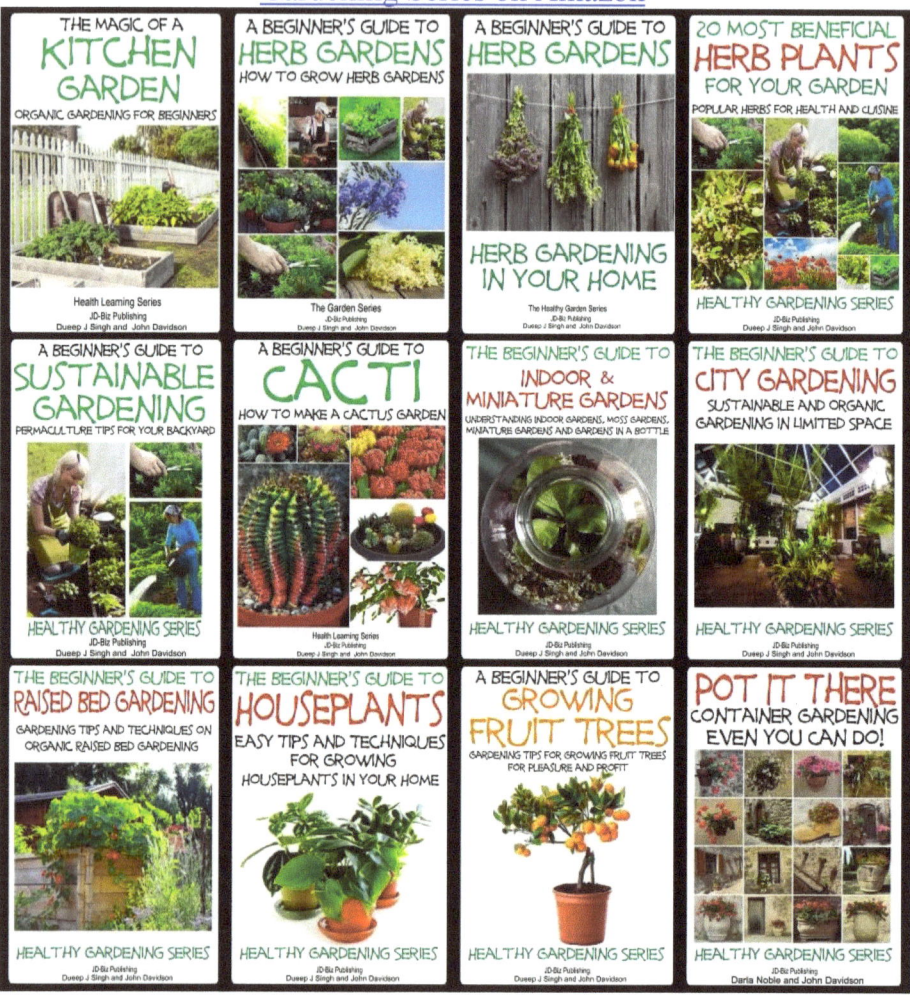

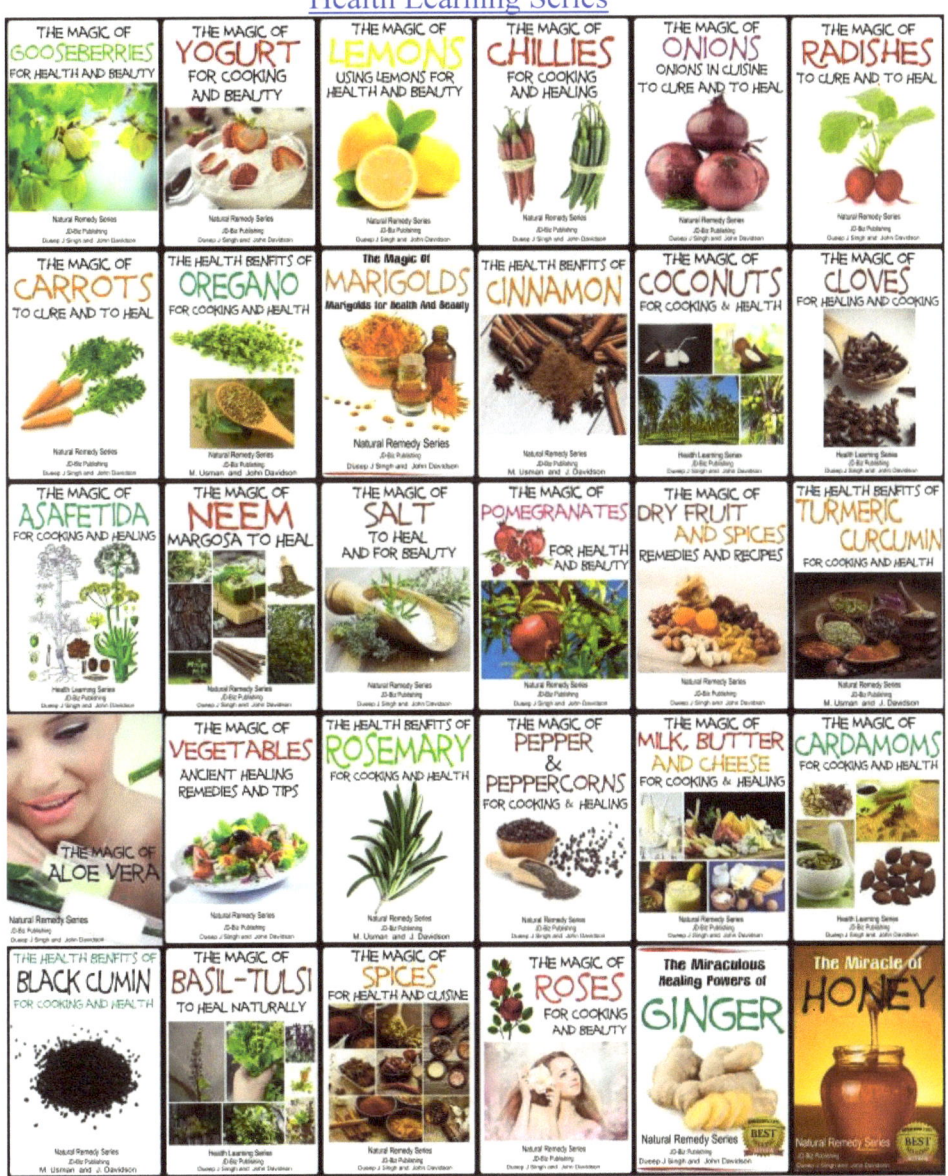

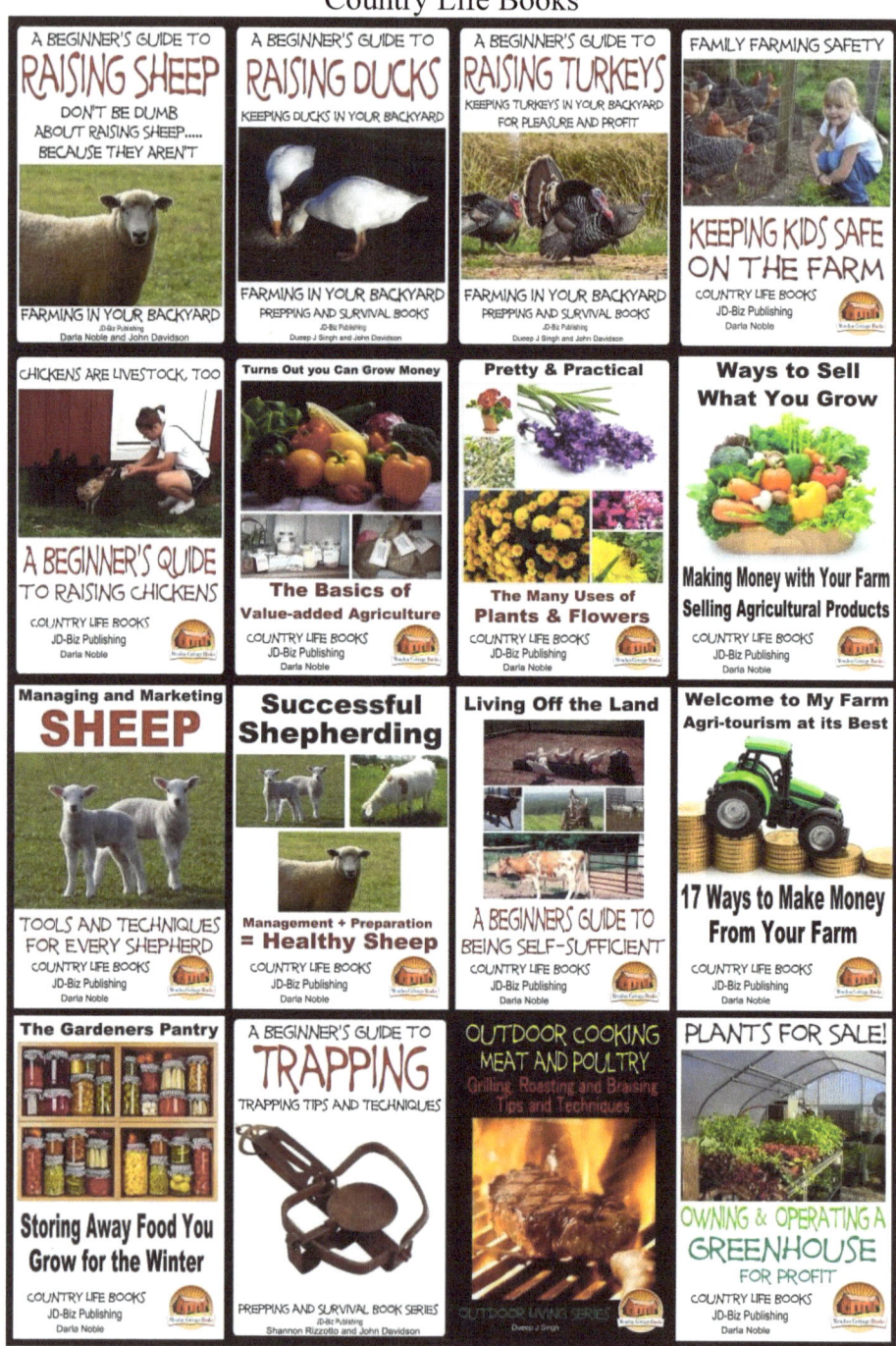

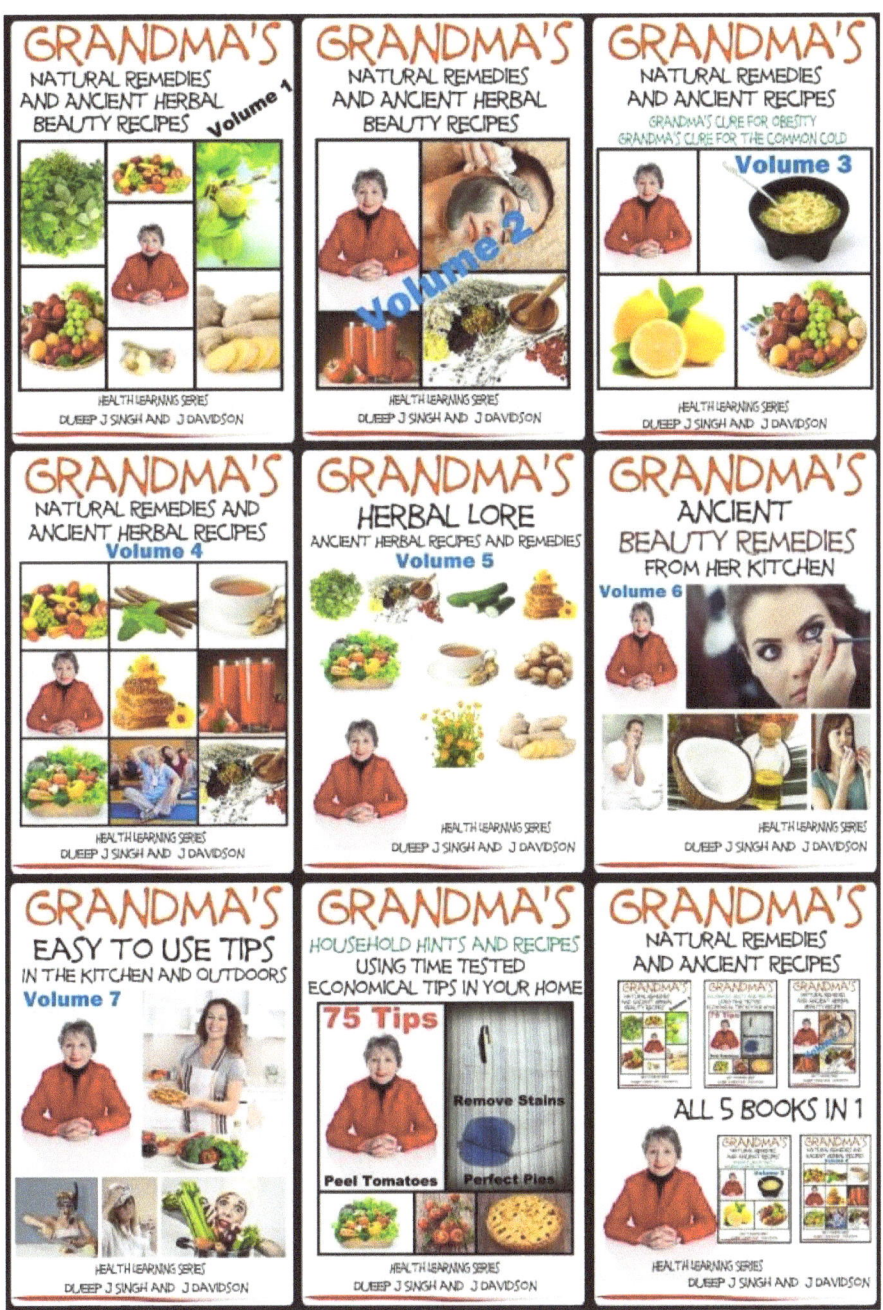

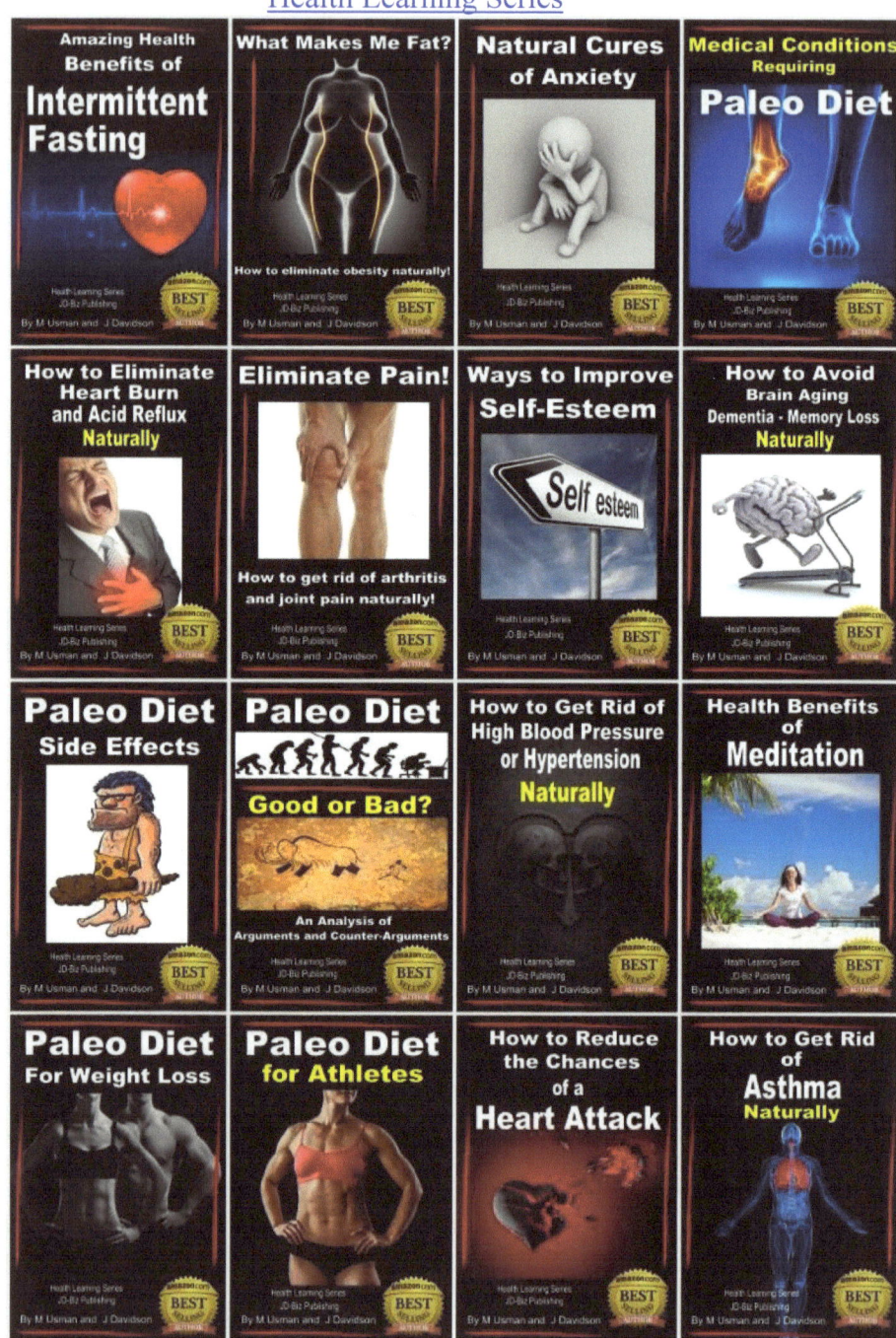

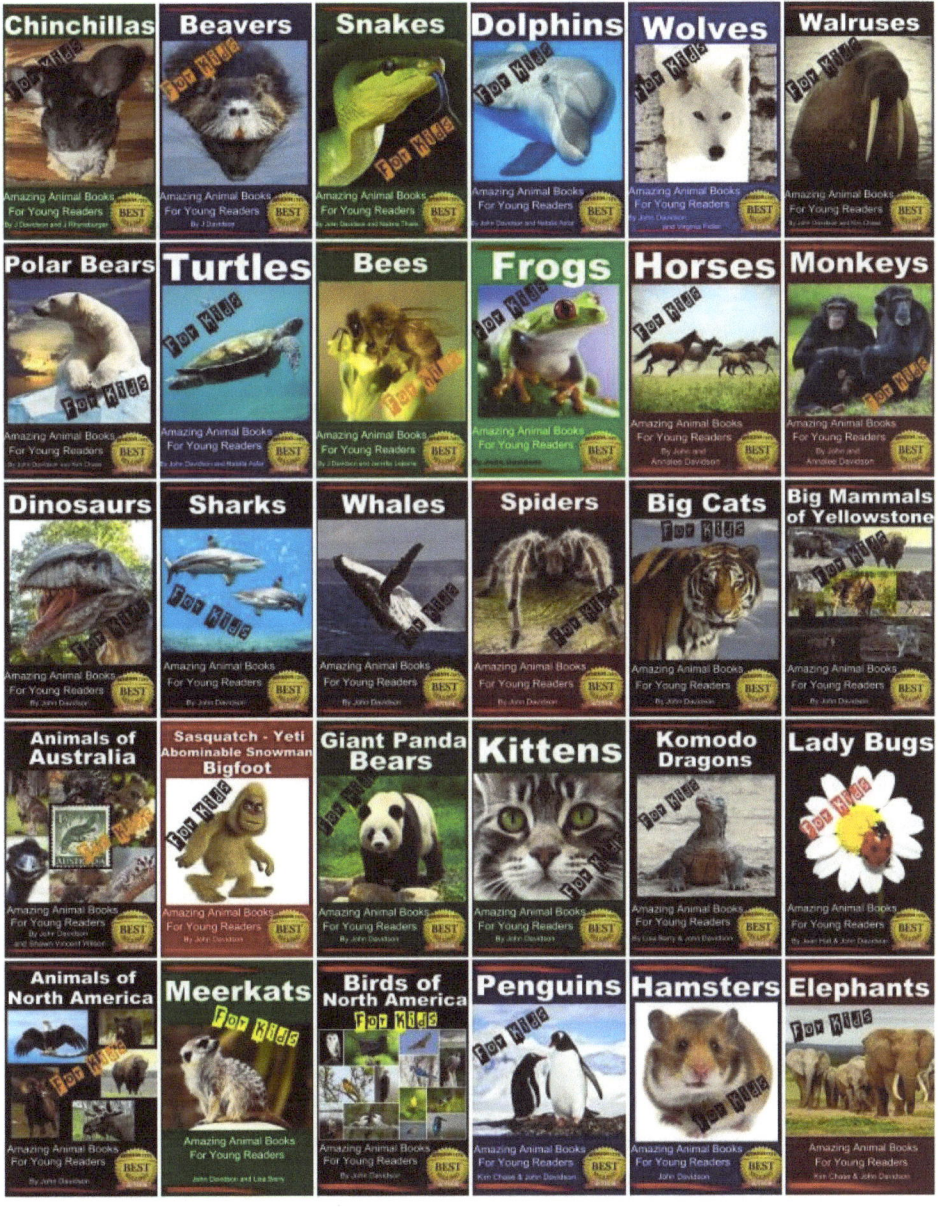

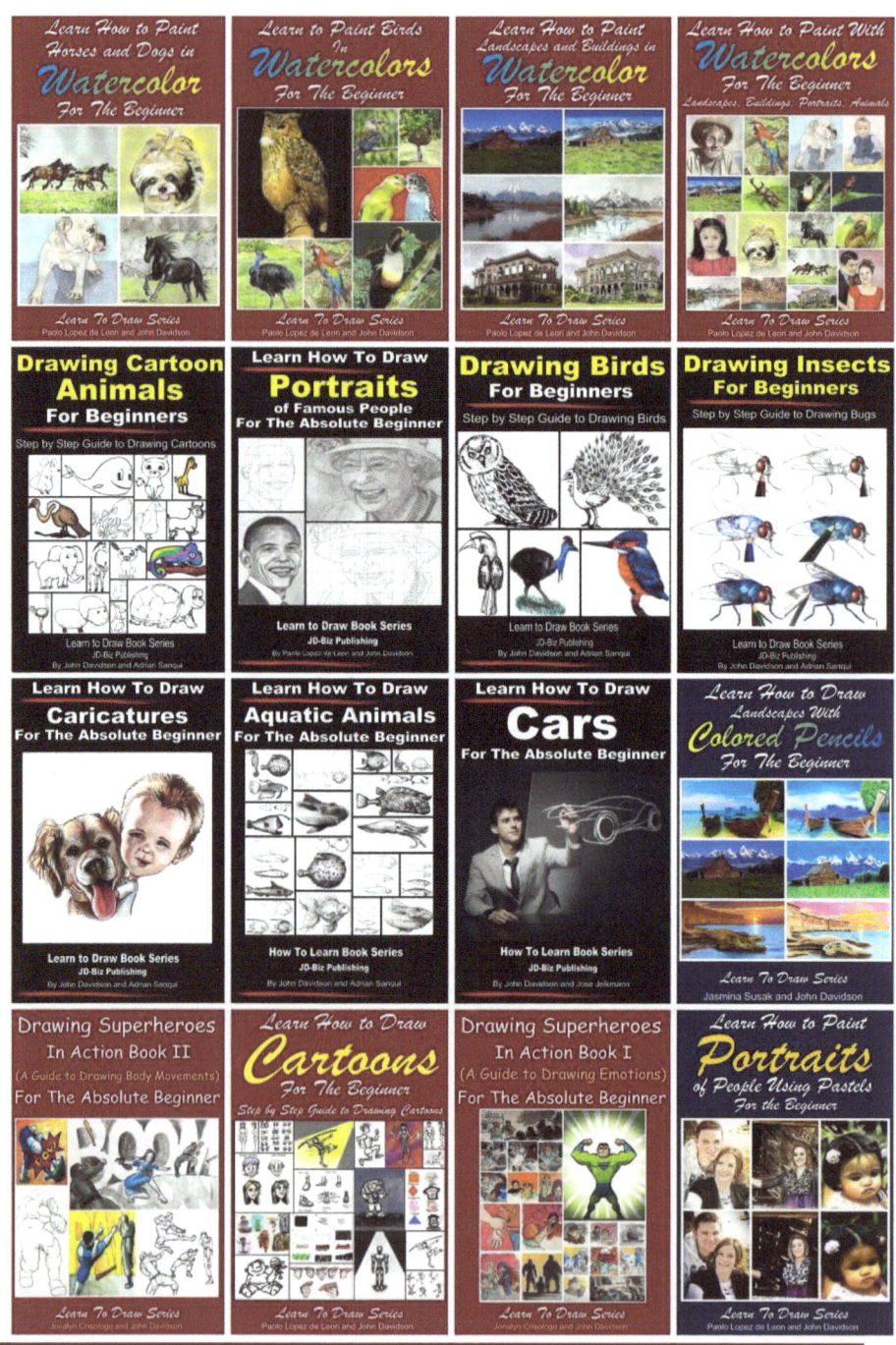

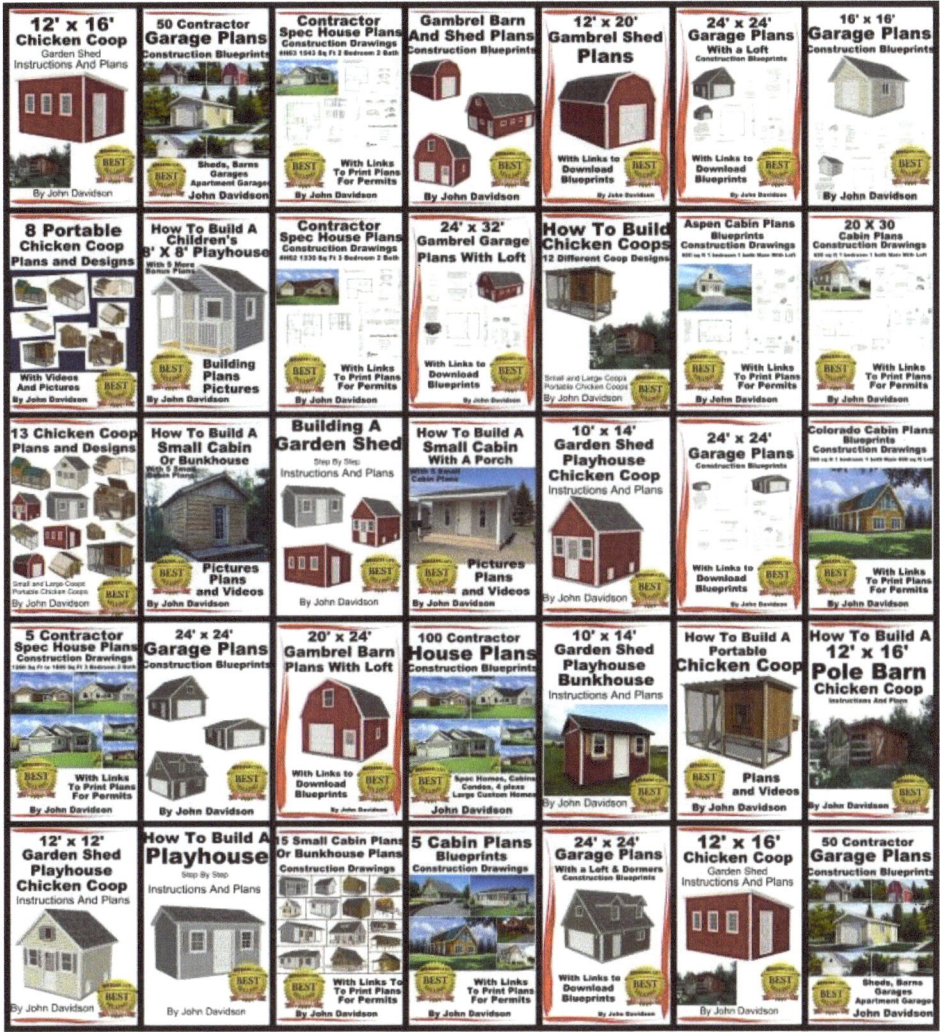

Entrepreneur Book Series

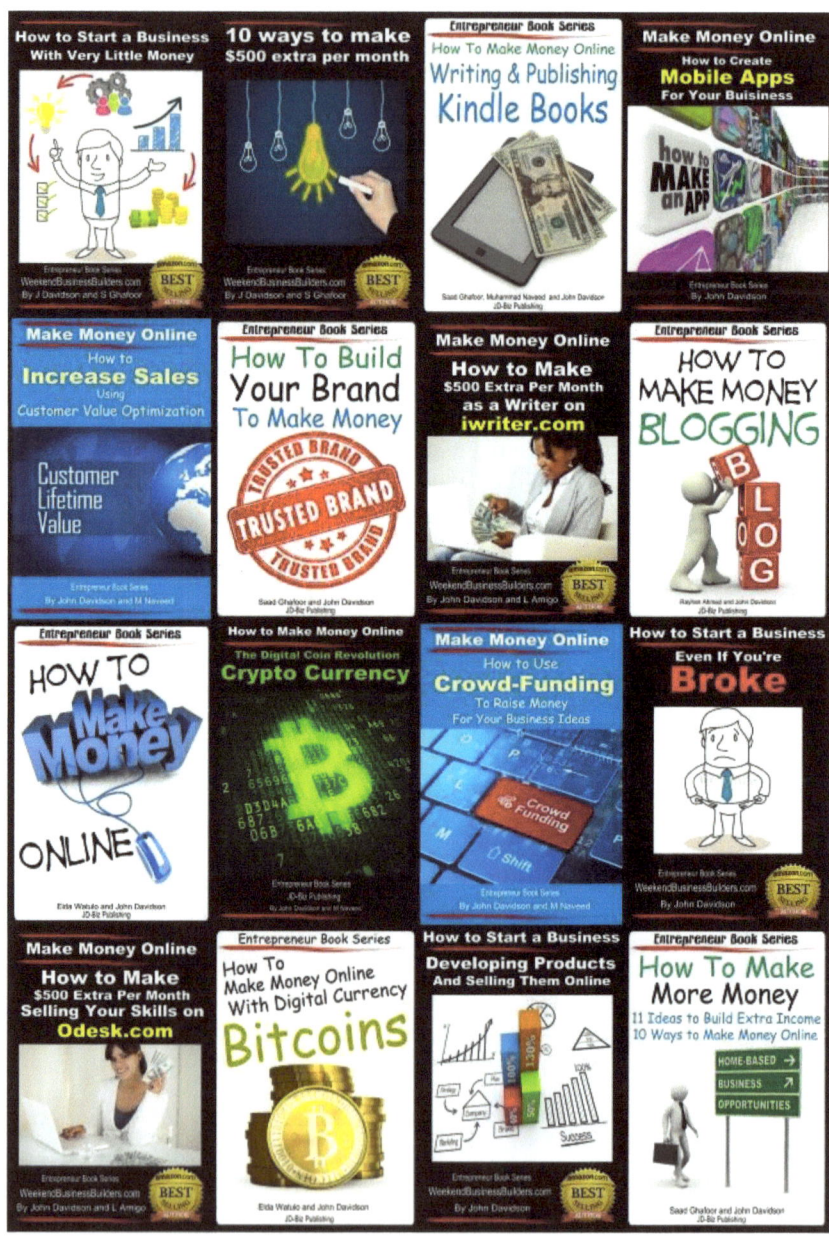

Our books are available at

1. Amazon.com
2. Barnes and Noble
3. Itunes
4. Kobo
5. Smashwords
6. Google Play Books

Download Free Books!

http://MendonCottageBooks.com

Publisher

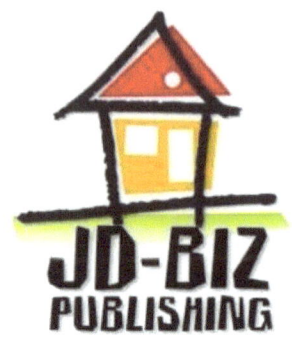

JD-Biz Corp

P O Box 374

Mendon, Utah 84325

http://www.jd-biz.com/

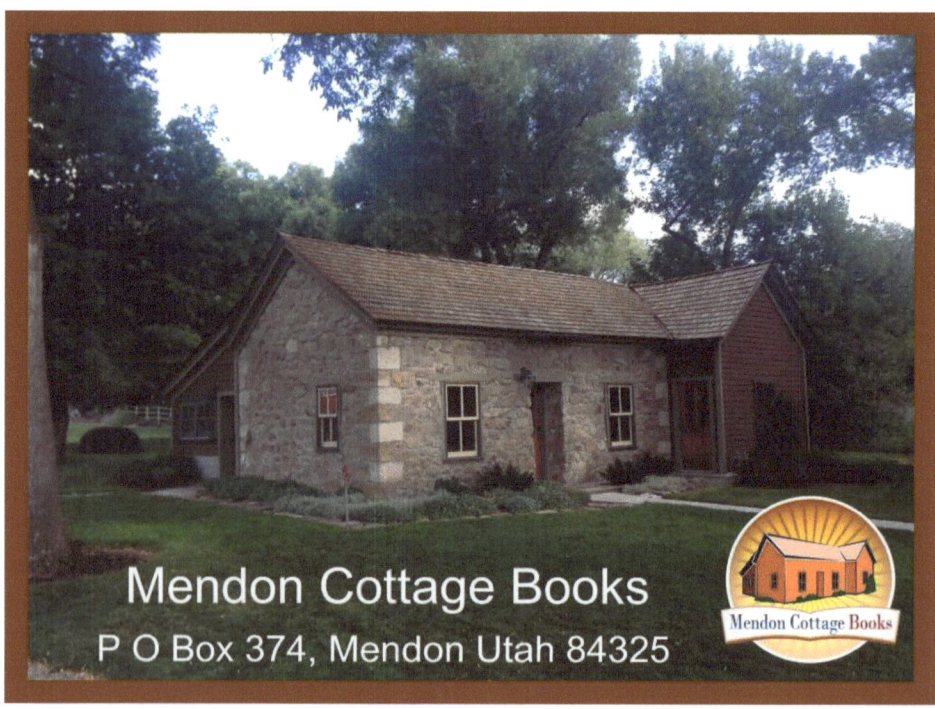

Mendon Cottage Books

P O Box 374, Mendon Utah 84325

www.ingramcontent.com/pod-product-compliance
Lightning Source LLC
Chambersburg PA
CBHW040313010626
45792CB00022B/289